SCIATICA
RELIEF NOW

Dean Volk PT

SCIATICA
RELIEF NOW

I Helped My Wife Overcome Excruciating SCIATICA

— Now It's Your Turn —

Dean Volk PT

Copyright © 2018 Dean Volk

All rights reserved. No part of this publication may be reproduced, stored in a retrieval system, or transmitted, in any form or in any means – by electronic, mechanical, photocopying, recording or otherwise – without prior written permission.

ISBN: 9781790277469

Acknowledgements

1. My amazing wife Trudy, whose support, painful story -- which you will read later, endless reading of my run-on sentences and constant encouragement has made me follow my dreams and pursue life as never before. Forever grateful to you!
2. Ben and Jesse – My two sons who always inspire me, encourage me and challenge me to be a better husband, dad and man. Love you two more than I know how to express!
3. Tom Dalonzo-Baker – Founder of Total Motion Release, the treatment technique I use most often and teach my clients in order for them to help themselves
4. Paul Gough and his amazing Media team – Amy Pope, Rachel Masshedar, Simon Godding, Sophie Gill, Rebecca Watson, Cameron Storer, Joe Walker and Vicki Smith. You have all inspired me, pushed me, taught me and driven me forward in pursuing my dreams. Thanks Coach and team!
5. My incredible staff at Volk Physical Therapy who have run my clinics with excellence. You have allowed me the time to pursue other ventures and dreams. Thank YOU!!
6. All my past clients, especially those who suffered with Sciatica or Piriformis syndrome. You have ALL been a contributor to this book as you were all my "guinea pigs" so-to-speak, that I got to practice all these techniques with and learn what does and does not work ☺.

CONTENTS

Introduction: Who Am I And Why I Have Written This Book ...1

Preface: [Take A Journey With Me] 9

Chapter 1: – Here They Are – The Three Best
Sciatica/Piriformis Syndrome Exercises 13

Chapter 2: Why These Exercises Work 25

Chapter 3: What Is Sciatica Anyway? 29

Chapter 4: What Is Priformis Syndrome? 31

Chapter 5: The 3 Most Common Causes Of Back Pain
And Sciatica 33

Chapter 6: Helpful Tips 37

A Final Note 47

About the Author 49

vii

INTRODUCTION
WHO AM I AND WHY I HAVE WRITTEN THIS BOOK

Hey there, my name is Dean Volk and I am a husband to an amazing wife for over 27 years, a father of two incredible young men, a physical therapy business owner for over 12 years, an international sciatica consultant and finally, now, a published author. I've been a Physical Therapist for over 26 years and I have cared for many clients who suffer from Sciatica and Piriformis Syndrome (PS). If you are reading this book, I am assuming you or a loved one has one of these issues (or you are my mom just wanting to see what I am up to!). The very first thing I want to convey to you is this: there is HOPE. I say this because I have two clinics in the Charlotte, NC area along with a concierge Mobile PT practice in Charleston, SC, and I have literally watched hundreds of clients through the years go from saying "there is no hope to beat this" or "this is probably the worst case you have ever dealt with" or "nothing has worked and I have tried everything" to absolute disbelief at the simple things which helped them turn their lives around. I love getting people out of pain, but more importantly, getting them back to living their lives and returning to doing the things they love without fear!

For those of you who may not know what a Physical Therapist is or does, I will briefly explain. First and foremost a Physical Therapist is a licensed professional which requires a post graduate degree, before passing national board exams. PT's are musculoskeletal experts that treat people with numerous conditions including: neck, shoulder, back, hip, knee ankle and foot issues. There are specialists who deal with hands, pediatric issues, women's health, orthopedic, and neurological issues. Over many years of treating patients, I have had the incredible privilege of watching people move from debilitating pain which had been present for days or years, to gaining their life back and returning to normal function. I honestly get a charge watching people overcome issues and return to doing what they love: which is why I felt compelled to write this book.

COMMON RECOMMENDATIONS FOR BACK PAIN ISSUES

I have been practicing physical therapy for a long time. I have seen many conditions and plenty of back pain syndromes including Sciatica and Piriformis problems. While treating Sciatica and Piriformis issues, I have heard some common recommendations given to my clients for these particular conditions.

Following are some of those recommendations:

"There isn't anything that can be done for this issue"

"You need only rest and medication to heal this condition"

"Surgery is your best (or only) option"

"You have a herniated (or bulging or protruding) disc and ONLY surgery will be able help you".

Now, there are well meaning and wonderful people who are working hard to help bring healing, and there are times when surgery IS required. However, there are times when healing can take place without surgery. In fact, recent studies are now revealing many surgical procedures are no more beneficial than doing nothing, and have many times made pain worse than when it first began.

WHAT LED ME HERE?

I could say my wife led me here but this would only be half of the story. What originally led me to want to help people heal from back pain were the results I began to experience as I treated patients. I began to see so much success I began to think about how many people I might be able to reach. This led me to reach people on-line and next to write this book. What took place with my wife only re-affirmed my decision.

THE STRANGE EVENT
THAT HAPPENED NEXT

Here is the WEIRD part. Just after I began helping people from all over the world on-line through webinars and through a FB Sciatica and Piriformis Syndrome RELIEF group, my wife experienced several days of the worst pain she had ever experienced. If you have had back pain you know how this feels. It's the feeling of being in pain and never finding a state of relief, and so it began. It was late June 2018 my wife woke me up one morning complaining of horrific pain. She said she was unable to get out of bed due to pain "running from her left buttocks all the way to her foot." It took her ten minutes to roll out of bed groaning in agony with every slight movement and stand up, though she was hunched over and any attempt to move caused her to yelp in pain. She even refused my help, as any touch or assistance caused her to brace more, increasing her suffering. She shuffled ever so slowly to use the restroom and back into bed. As she lay there in agony, I literally said, "You cannot have Sciatica, I am an International Sciatica Consultant!" It turned out to be on of the longest days of her life, as she tried to find positions of comfort (even if for 30 seconds of relief), attempted slow moving gentle exercises, and doing all she could to avoid pain.

That night I was awakened by her moaning, "I don't know why I'm going through this! I don't know what I did! There is NO comfortable position! Nothing is helping! Why am I going through this!? I didn't do anything to cause this! It hurts all the way from my butt to my ankle! Any little movement is excruciating! I cannot find a comfortable position! I just need to get some sleep!" IF you have ever muttered these words YOU can relate!! And IF you have ever said these things about your sciatica—YOU are reading the right book, because I wrote this just for you. You understand what it is like to have shooting pains through your buttocks and leg with the slightest movement. You understand. Every breath makes you cringe in anticipation of the next severe, bone chilling shock. You are familiar with the agony of brushing your teeth, shifting your hips in bed and doing any simple daily activity we all take for granted. IF you can relate to thinking and feeling these things, then this book is for YOU.

Needless to say, that night terrible for my wife, but thankfully, each night thereafter was much improved. It took 3-4 days for her to start moving semi-comfortably for short durations. She began standing upright, being able to slowly do a few normal activities. By day 7 she was walking 2-3 miles with shortened step lengths to avoid stressing the Sciatic Nerve. There were minor set-backs with short durations of intense pain, but they grew further and further apart and became less and less intense. By day 10, she was functioning normally and just using ice as a precaution to avoid any undue inflammation.

My wife, made an amazingly full recovery within about 10 days and as her Physical Therapist, I made certain we were cautious NOT to overdo anything, since she was feeling almost too good! So—what made the difference for her as compared to what most people go through? It was the fact that I knew which exercises and motions she could do, and what she should avoid. We attacked it early and consistently, we avoided movement and painful positions as much as possible, focusing on positions and motions of comfort − even if she only held it for 15 seconds before having to search for another position to ease the pain. We did try some Hemp Oil, but it aggravated her stomach. She had NO pain meds, NO injections, NO MRIs or tests. She has slight stenosis, which we have known, but over all we did nothing more than proper positioning, motions/exercises and a good old-fashioned ice pack, with a Salonpas (Lidocaine) patch or two. Was she lucky? OR, was it because we got right on it and knew what to do? Plus, she was consistent and faithful to the routine and the results speak for themselves.

After looking back and going through this personally, I truly feel even more strongly, I have something to offer people, using a unique approach as compared to what I was reading throughout the web. So, I continued with my on-line group and individual patients with a bit more fervor. This incident woke me up. I had been helping clients for years, but this was my wife, and I really wanted her out of pain. I wanted her out of pain fast and I put everything I knew to practice. I further came to realize I could help people during their time of distress and totally empathize and relate to their situations more directly than ever before. I also came to realize what I am doing is exactly what I am supposed to be doing – helping people like YOU.

IMAGINE WHAT YOU COULD DO WITHOUT BACK PAIN

Before I go further, I want you to think of some questions for your own life. Imagine YOUR pain and agony eliminated within a week's time! Go ahead and let your mind think of what you really want to do again. What would you be doing right now IF you were able? What are YOU NOT doing right now out of fear of flaring your sciatica symptoms? These questions are important ones to consider as you navigate your health and consider how you want to handle your problem. The pains and frustrations caused by Sciatica and Piriformis Syndrome can truly undermine your daily living. I personally get much joy out of helping others redeem their lives and have hope again. Watching someone pick up their grandchildren; get back to riding a bike; running again, playing golf for the first time in months and just enjoying life again are all things that bring me true joy. Because of this, I have dedicated much of my life studying the facts, as well as the best methods to help heal these syndromes.

PREFACE

[TAKE A JOURNEY WITH ME]
A Quick Run-Down of Back Pain Statistics and Why I Wrote This Book

BEFORE I WRITE about the treatments I use for Sciatica and Piriformis issues, I thought I would give some quick facts and statistics about back pain. I have read statistics that show low back pain is the #1 reason for days missed from work in America. 80% of Americans will suffer low back pain at least 1x in their life. MOST people will not seek medical attention initially for low back pain, and for those who do, only 4-6% of them will be sent to a Physical Therapist for help. Studies show that IF a person undergoes an MRI for their back pain, before seeing a Physical Therapist, they will typically spend $4500+ more on their care, compared to those who see a Physical Therapist first. I could go on and on, but needless to say, back pain is a huge issue not just from a pain perspective, but it affects a person financially, mentally and emotionally.

Because I have a passion for helping people, it hit

me one day – What if I could write a reasonably short, easy-to-read book which could give some quick and to-the-point answers? I thought, 'what if I could help people by explaining **WHAT** exercises they can do in their own home and explain the **REASONING** behind these exercises so they could obtain an amount of relief?' Sod, here you are reading it….NO one likes to live on pain medications or depend on drugs day-in and day- out, and not many people I know love the thought of a possible surgery. For those reasons, I wrote this book -- to offer hope and show there could be a better way!! Please enjoy the book. And, IF you have ANY questions, feel free to reach out to me at info@SciaticaReliefNow.net.

FIRST LET'S GET YOU OUT OF PAIN
The end of the book first

Why not give you the information you need to know right away?! Anyone who knows me knows I am the type of person who likes to get to the bottom line quickly. I like results and I like to be able to fix a problem in the simplest and most efficient manner. So, I wrote this book with this in mind. I strategically set it up differently than most. I decided to give you the methods FIRST so that I could relieve your pain as quickly as possible. I also decided to add pictures so you can see how to do these exercises.

After the methods, IF you would like to understand the WHY and the WHAT you will find those answers at the END of this book. In essence, I wrote this book BACKWARDS. I don't get into the REASONS first, I give the RESULTS first because time is short. If I can get YOU out of initial pain as soon as possible then I am doing my job. I've also included a few helpful tips for your daily living to prevent injury and aid in your healing.

CHAPTER 1

– HERE THEY ARE –
THE THREE BEST SCIATICA/ PIRIFORMIS SYNDROME EXERCISES

F OR THOSE PEOPLE who suffer with Sciatica, there IS good news! I have three very simple exercises, which I have used over the past 12+ years which can ease your symptoms in minutes. If you are suffering from Sciatica or Piriformis Syndrome, on ONE side of the body only, these three exercises WILL prove to be amazingly helpful to control, and often times eliminate your pain. People from around the WORLD are using these exercises to get relief quickly and easily.

RULES FOR MY EXERCISES OR ACTIVITIES:

1. **If any activity causes pain, discomfort or soreness while performing -- STOP.**

2. **ONLY perform activities to the Looser, More comfortable and Less restricted side or "LML."**
3. **If the exercise or activity you just performed had a positive result on your symptoms, do it again!**

These movements can give quick and sometimes long-lasting relief when performed correctly. One thing to keep in mind is these exercises may need to be repeated frequently to combat long-standing issues. You may wonder at first, why you are doing what you are doing, but trust me and stick with it. I will explain the "why" at the end of this book.

EXERCISE 1

THE TWIST

PLEASE REMEMBER THE acronym "LML" = **L**ooser, **M**ore Comfortable Movement, **L**ess Restricted.

1. While seated at the edge of a chair or bed, twist to your right and then to your left as far as you can each way. Determine which side is the LML or basically, which way does your body like to turn better?
2. Choose the LML side to perform 2 sets of 25 twists.

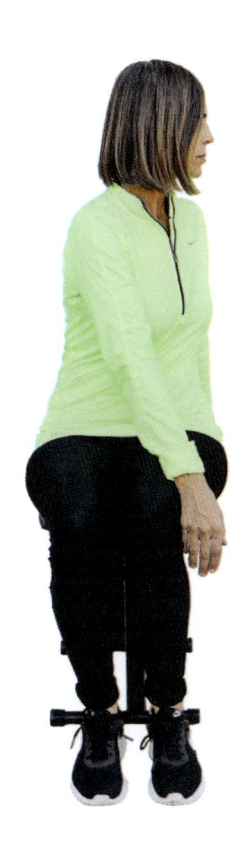

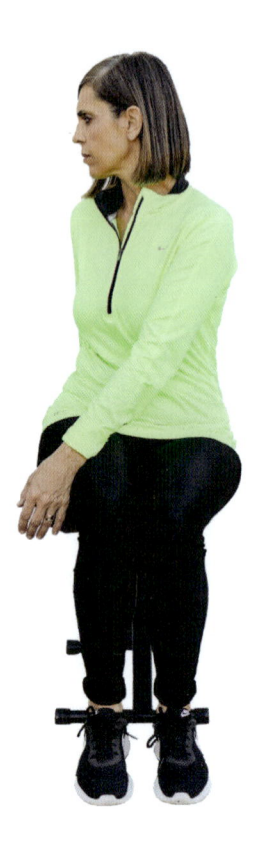

3. When completed, retest the twist to the other side (to see IF there is any change in movement, tightness, or pain). Also, assess YOUR symptoms (whether it be back, butt, hip or leg pain).

4. If anything from #3 above improves, REPEAT 2 more sets of these twists to the same side as above. Repeat steps 2-3 above, until there is no more improvement of symptoms or symptoms are eliminated.

Each of these activities will follow the same pattern.
1. Test (to find LML)
2. Exercise
3. Retest opposite side movement 4. Assess YOUR symptoms.

Dean Volk PT

EXERCISE 2

THE PIRIFORMIS STRETCH

ANOTHER SIMPLE, YET effective activity is the Piriformis Stretch (see pictures below -can be done seated or lying on your back, whichever is more comfortable for you). Once again, do as you did with the above exercise:

1. While seated or lying down, stretch as shown below, first the right side, then the left. Determine which side is the LML (IF piriformis syndrome, your painful side WILL cause pain).

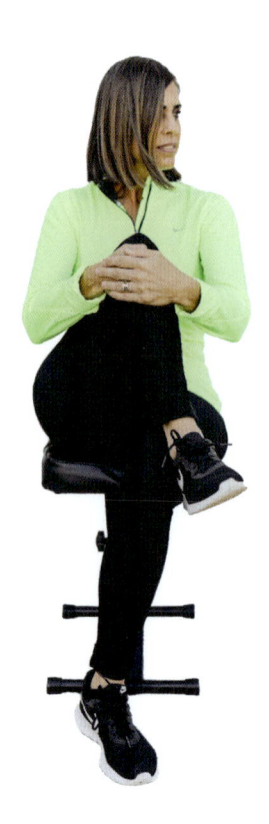

OR

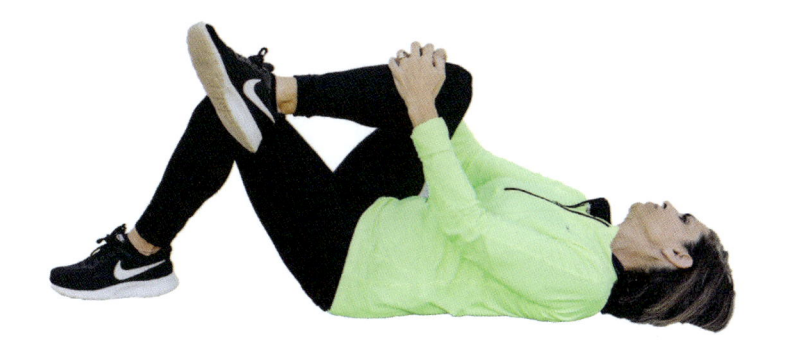

2. Choose the LML side to perform exercise by pulling the knee, toward the opposite shoulder, as shown above. Hold this stretch for 30 seconds, repeat 10x

3. When completed, retest the stretch to the other side (to see IF there is any change in movement, tightness, or pain). Also, assess YOUR symptoms (whether it be back, butt, hip or leg pain

4. If anything from #3 above improves, REPEAT stretch another 10x, to same side as #2 above. Repeat steps 2-3 above, until there is no more improvement of symptoms, or symptoms are eliminated.

I typically see relief of 50-80% of the severe intense pain with these two simple exercises. On a rare occasion these two exercises do NOT afford relief. If you are among those without relief, do NOT worry there is more to come!

EXERCISE 3

THE STRAIGHT LEG RAISE

THIS SIMPLE EXERCISE is designed to find differences/ restrictions or pain while comparing right and left sides. With Sciatica one usually has a painful leg. To test pain levels, do the following: Again, remember the acronym "LML"

1. Sit on the edge of a chair (or bed) and straighten one leg so the heel is on the floor, and attempt to lift that leg straight into the air, as pictured below: (keeping the knee as straight as possible) You will compare right side to left side as in the previous two exercises to determine the LML side.

WARNING: Often people with sciatica get pain just trying to extend their heel to the floor, before lifting their leg upwards, IF that is the case **DO NOT LIFT** the leg.

Sciatica Relief Now

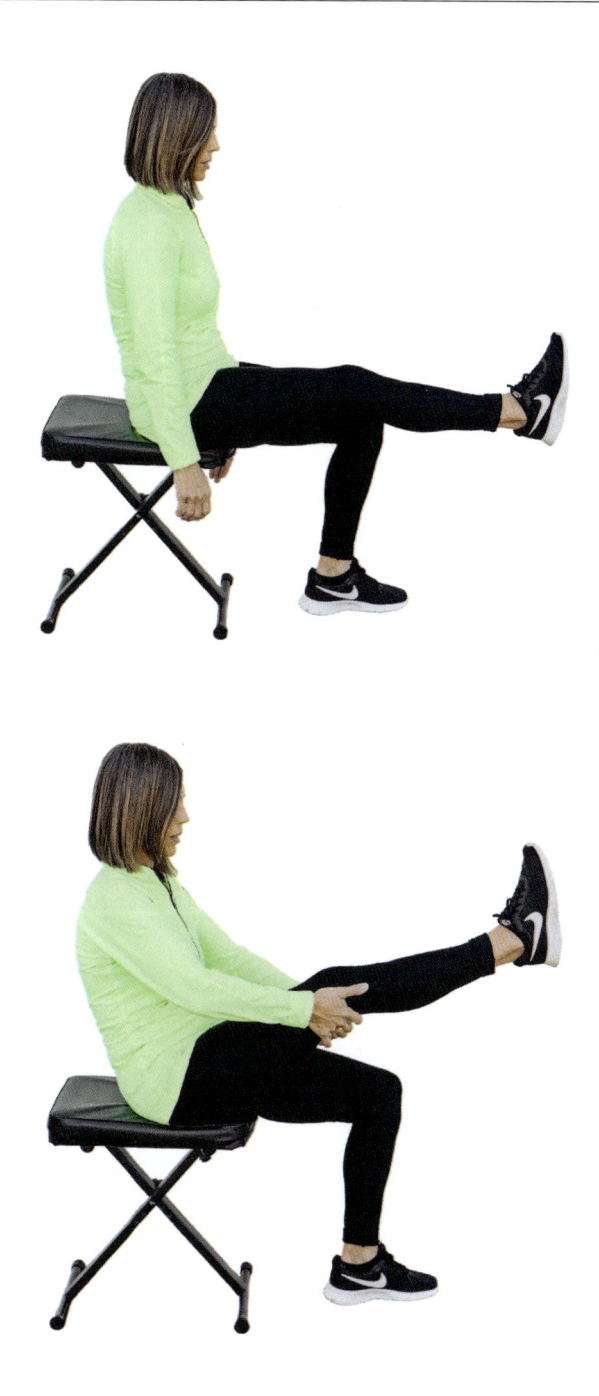

2. Choose the LML side to perform exercise by using your arms to hold your leg, behind your knee, with both hands. Lift with your arms and LML side leg, until you feel a pull in the back of the leg. Lift as high as you comfortably can. Then "bounce" the leg at its highest position 25x then relax and repeat a 2nd set.
3. When completed, retest the leg lift to the other side (to see IF there is any change in movement, tightness, or pain). Also, assess YOUR symptoms (whether it be back, butt, hip or leg pain
4. If anything from #3 above improves, REPEAT bouncing the same leg as above 2 sets of 25 reps. Repeat steps 2-3 above, until there is no more improvement of symptoms, or symptoms are eliminated.

COMPLETE TREATMENT AND CARE

Although these exercises can offer good relief of symptoms it is not likely these activities will completely "fix" your underlying problem. Getting out of initial pain begins the first step on your Road to Recovery. I suggest you perform these exercises a minimal of 2x a day, or as often as needed to calm down pain.

For a complete recovery program, I would suggest finding out more of what I offer at www.SciaticaReliefNow.net. Or, if you have a trusted Physical Therapist in your local area who specializes in low back and Sciatica issues, see them for a complete back program. These exercises are a great start, and may leave some therapists scratching their heads. Not many Physical Therapists use this technique I've just written about to help their clients. This form of treatment is called **Total Motion Release**

(TMR), a technique developed by Tom Dalonzo-Baker from Raleigh, NC. Find more information at totalmotionrelease.com. Having been a therapist for 25+ years, I have NOT found any one technique which works so consistently, with such profound results. Here are just a few quotes from clients I have treated throughout my years of practice.

BERNIE, NORTH CAROLINA

"I've been suffering with Sciatica for the last 2 years and been going to a chiropractor, after the last year it hasn't worked. I came to Dean and he has put me into Total Motion Release Therapy. I've been on the road to recovery since then and it's been great."

BRITTANY, IN CALIFORNIA

"I had a video conference call with Dean last Friday. I was skeptical what I could possibly learn over a video conference that I had not already learned from my physical therapist or doctors. Well… I learned a lot! He stressed to me that focusing your energy on stretching and doing body movements on your good side will in turn help release tight muscles like your piriformis on your bad side. I had been experiencing sciatica for the last 1.5 years. He taught me a few very valuable stretches that have improved my sciatic pain by approximately 50% already. I plan to continue doing the stretches on a regular basis and I am finally feeling optimistic about getting rid of this sciatic pain for good. He provided me information that no other doctors or physical therapist had taught me. If you are living with sciatica on a regular basis I would highly recommend that you speak with Dean! "

ANDREW, IN GREAT BRITAIN

"Your help and videos etc (over the past several weeks) have been more than what I've received from the NHS in the 12 years I've been back in this country since leaving the Army. "

NICK, A PT IN FLORIDA

"I am a physical therapist and have tried every trick/exercise under the sun and was not able to get relief from my Sciatica and Back Pain! None of the conventional stuff that is used by standard therapists or chiropractors worked! I was really starting to LOSE HOPE. Was I not fixable? At times I would just HOPE that it would go away and it never did! For 5 Years I had dealt with Sciatica and Low Back Pain. In 30 minutes of working with Dean I FINALLY got the relief that I wanted and now am confident that I can play with my kids, sit, lay down, and be active again WITHOUT worrying about my Sciatica holding me back. I even learned the exact technique that Dean uses, and I STILL couldn't fix myself. The problem was I wasn't doing it RIGHT. Dean helped tweak what I was doing and BOOM! INSTANT RELIEF! Thanks Dean! (I was SUPER SKEPTICAL at first and worried he couldn't help me because I had tried so much before.......but he delivered as promised!)"

LORRAINE, IN UK

"The only relief I get from this awful pain is by doing Deans exercises every day and as needed. I'm on extremely strong pain killers for other illnesses and they do not touch it! I'm talking Morphine, Tramadol Kapake! When you get that relief after the exercises it is wonderful! So do please try them"

CHAPTER 2
WHY THESE EXERCISES WORK

Now that you have tried these exercises, let me explain the reason why they work. In actuality, it's a pretty simple reason. Think of what happens to your car when you have a tire blow-out. The structure of the car gets off "balance" and there is abnormal tension throughout the car's frame. This becomes realized by a strong pull through the steering column as the driver attempts to control the car. Even though the car is off-kilter, the frame of the car is still solid. However, imagine what would happen IF the frame was not solid. Imagine if it had multiple moving joints, with thick rubber bands wrapped around those joints. Are you following me? In order to alleviate the unnatural tension, the joints would move, and shift and those rubber bands would be stressed, stretched, shortened, and put into abnormal and unfamiliar positions.

BODY COMPENSATION

Now, for a moment, think of your body as the car frame but without being a solid piece of immovable steel, think of it with joints, and rubber bands. When injured, your body (like the car) strains, moves and adjusts itself in any way possible to avoid the pain, which causes it to become imbalanced (compared to normal). Here's a simple example of what happens when the body experiences a pain or strain. Let's look at when you sprain your right ankle for example. What affect does this have on your right knee, on your right hip, and on your low back? Also, how does it affect your left ankle, your left knee or your left hip? How is the now present limp affecting your walking? Are your shoulders swinging in their normal pattern when you walk? Do you see where I am going with all of this? Our body is an amazing piece of equipment. It is built with intricate interrelationships and interdependence upon every other part of itself. Our bodies are masters at "compensating" for pain, adapting to soreness, pain, tightness and any other restriction which comes its way. When our body faces any type of pain, stiffness, tightness, soreness or discomfort for any reason, I like to point clients back to the blown tire analogy. Because our body is stressed like a car frame, no matter how intensely or subtly, our entire body is affected. Knowing this, you can realize when any type of stress in the body occurs, our normal balanced body, gets "out of balance" from right to left side. Does this make sense so far??

THE PAINFUL SIDE

Now, you can see pain, stiffness, tightness, soreness or discomfort can cause the body to naturally compensate throwing your balance off right side to left side. Knowing this, would it make sense to try to move a painful body part any more than necessary? IF the painful part is moved, the body will compensate for the pain which will further aggravate the imbalance of your body? Can you see that it would throw you further out of balance?

GETTING YOUR BODY BACK IN BALANCE

SO, what is the answer? How do you get your body back in balance? How do you avoid the painful motions and alleviate symptoms? Hopefully, you did just that with the Sciatica exercises above. IF you are not a Sciatica sufferer, and just reading this book for knowledge sake, the answer is simply this: Move the body parts that are **NOT** painful, tight, sore, or uncomfortable. Yes, I KNOW this sounds strange, but I'll write it again: Move the UN-painful, UN-restricted, UN-sore, and comfortable side. Move the '**good** side.' Remember my acronym – "LML" … **L**ooser, **M**ore Comfortable, **L**ess Restrictive? Well, this is the "WHY" behind that initial instruction. What does this accomplish? As strange as this might sound, this type of movement allows your body to relax. It actually eases tension and allows the body to move comfortably. This also creates an amazing calming effect on the painful, stiff, tight and sore areas of your body. As a child of the 60's (a very, very young child), I can still remember a common theme of that decade, **"IF it feels good do it!"** Well, this actually applies amazingly well in this scenario. Move the good side. If it feels good move it.

This is the reason I have my Sciatica clients, from chapter 1, twist to their looser side, stretch their more comfortable buttock/hip and lift their less restricted leg. Because --**#1**, IF we exercised the painful side, it would cause further stress and imbalance in our bodies and

#2 because it is MUCH more comfortable to exercise the side that feels good and is easier to move than the bad side! This may sound strange but, I have acheived faster results working the good side. I have also noticed my clients are much more likely to follow directions when things are NOT painful to do. This allows the client to focus on simple pain free motions which reduces stress, anxiety, and pain which accompanies working the painful side.

CHAPTER 3
WHAT IS SCIATICA ANYWAY?

Sciatica is a generic name for any symptomatic condition that involves the Sciatic nerve. The nerve is made up of five nerve roots which come from your lower back and join together to travel through the buttocks, down the back of the leg, splits into 2 nerves behind the knee, which then travels to the foot. Sciatica is a condition in which the Sciatic Nerve is compromised, whether by a spasming muscle, a bulging or herniated disc in the low back, a compression in the spine, or any type of irritation of the nerve along its route. It is most commonly caused by pressure against the nerve. Symptoms can vary greatly and range from sharp searing pains to a dull ache, burning sensations to numbness, tingling sensations as well as loss of strength in the muscles the nerve controls. Pains and symptoms are most commonly noted in the buttock, middle of hamstring muscle or in the calf. It is NOT uncommon to have pains or symptoms radiating all the way to the foot. Symptoms can vary day to day, in intensity, in type of symptoms as well as locations of those symptoms, depending on activities, positions and what is actually causing the sciatica.

One important consideration which seems to be consistent with Sciatica is this the sooner it is treated properly, the quicker the recovery time and the best chance to minimize any possible damage. Too often, people ignore initial symptoms thinking they will go away on their own. My encouragement to you is to get help as fast as possible to minimize damage which can shorten recovery time.

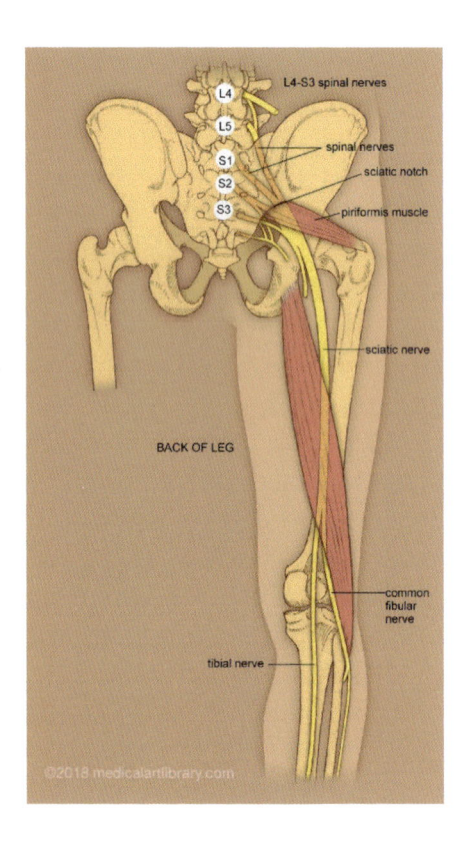

CHAPTER 4
WHAT IS PRIFORMIS SYNDROME?

SIMPLY PUT, PIRIFORMIS Syndrome (PS), is closely related to sciatica, due to the proximity of the Piriformis Muscle to the Sciatic Nerve in the center of the buttocks. Studies show that the Sciatic Nerve ~80% of time it runs below the muscle. In 5-10% of people the nerve runs above the muscle. In 10-15% it pierces through the muscle belly. If there is any irritation of Piriformis muscle [causing pain] whether due to an injury, muscle spasms, or tightness can be classified as Piriformis Syndrome. Symptoms always include significant buttock pain, with varying amounts of pain in hip and those symptoms are consistent with sciatica.

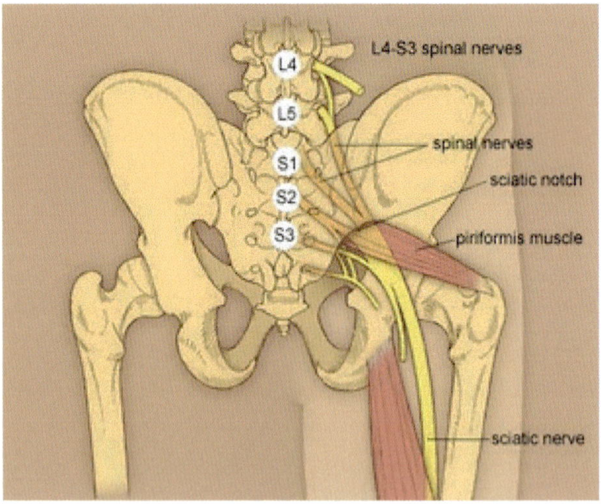
L4-S3 spinal nerves
L4
L5
S1
S2
S3
spinal nerves
sciatic notch
piriformis muscle
sciatic nerve

CHAPTER 5

THE 3 MOST COMMON CAUSES OF BACK PAIN AND SCIATICA

THE THREE MOST common causes of low back pain and sciatica are:

1. Herniated Disc
2. Stenosis (caused by degenerative disc disease (DDD) or arthritis)
3. SI Joint Dysfunction.

A herniated disc in the spine typically moves backwards towards the spinal nerve roots. If the bulge touches the nerve root(s), this can cause pain along the entire distribution of the nerve. Since the nerve roots form the nerves into the leg, pressure on these roots can cause pain all the way down the leg into the foot (tingling, burning and numbness well).

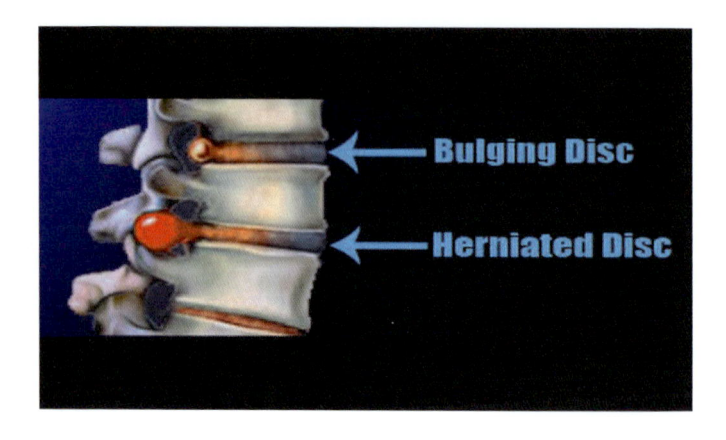

Stenosis simply means narrowing of the spine. This can be caused by several different

"degenerative" processes: degenerative disc disease (DDD), degenerative joint disease (DJD)

and other types of "wear and tear." Some people are even born with a certain amount of

stenosis. As the space around the spine narrows nerves can get pinched.

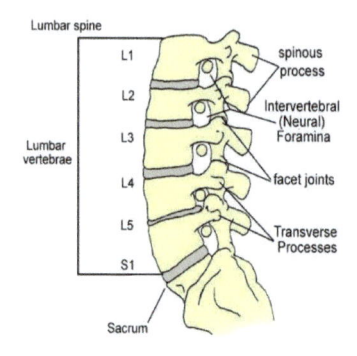

The SI joints are where your pelvis connects to your spine, the low back "dimples".

People with **SI** pain typically have pain they can touch when they push on the joints usually have buttocks tenderness as well.

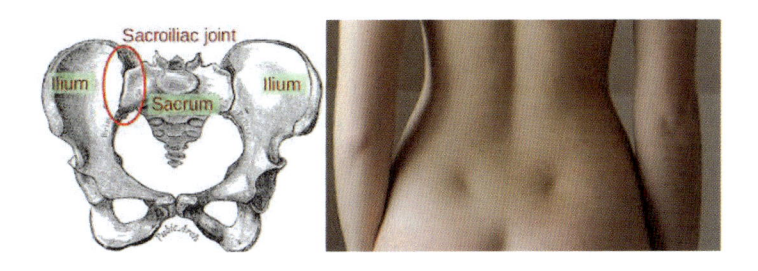

PAIN AT NIGHT

Why is pain more intense when you lie down at night rather than during the day? This is a common question which deserves an answer. Here are some of the reasons why pain is more intense during the night.

First of all, during the day there is an increased amount of stimulation going on with our senses. Our eyes open to see things; our ears hear many noises; we smell, taste and touch. All of these things stimulate our brain. Our senses actually bombard our brain with constant input and this can distract areas of our body which are experiencing pain. Obviously this can seem to be a good thing until we decide to head to bed.

When you lie down at night, typically, our senses calm down. Our brain is an amazing organ, available to receive an incredible amount of information. However, during the night as there are less sensory actions to our brain, there is less information being inputted, and the brain becomes less stimulated. As a result, the brain is undistracted, so it can focus toward the pain going on in our body. If you have a bit of pain during the day this pain may be magnified at night due to the fact the pain then becomes the primary input to your brain.

PAIN IN THE MORNING

Why is my pain more significant in the morning? Why does it take me a significant amount of time walking around to calm it down?

INFLAMMATION BUILD-UP

The answer here is you have inflammation build-up. As we sleep we tend to lie still. If there is any inflammation already taking place our body, this area becomes a bit stiff. As a result, the body is more stiff and achy in the morning. Moving our muscles helps reduce inflammation by increasing circulation. Think of it as motion it lotion to our body -- pumping out the inflammation.

IF the pain is a result of a disc issue, discs enlarge (very slightly) as we lie down for the night and do not have gravity compressing the disc. Our discs absorb water through the night and enlarge, which causes a bulge or herniation to enlarge as well. So, if a herniation is touching or compressing something causing pain, it is more compressed at night. Once we are up and around, the disc releases water due to the compression of the disc from gravity, which shrinks the disc. Here's a fun little side note: If you want to be taller—measure your height first thing in the morning!

CHAPTER 6
HELPFUL TIPS

SLEEPING TIPS

THERE ARE MANY benefits of getting good sleep. One of the more interesting facts is this: sleep reduces inflammation. In fact, sleep can be one of the strongest natural anti-inflammatory agents out there. Sleep can actually help reduce levels of inflammatory proteins in the blood, more specifically, the C-reactive protein. People who sleep under six hours have a higher risk of developing inflammatory conditions.

☆ MY BED OF CHOICE

My bed of choice is a sleep number bed. It can be expensive but the massive advantage is it can adapt to your needs. Since our bodies need change day to day, our bed should ideally do the same. This adjustable mattress can adapt to your body, so if you need a soft mattress one night, a firm or extra firm the next night, you can achieve your desired firmness with the sleep number bed by a push of a button.

☆ IF I AM IN PAIN, HOW SHOULD I POSITION MYSELF WHILE I SLEEP?

My preferential position for sleeping is side-lying 'bad-side' up with a pillow between the knees and the knees bent up in a not-so-tight fetal position. Other positions many find comfortable are either lying on your back with your head propped up slightly and a pillow underneath your knees or lying on your stomach with a pillow underneath your waist to keep spine from extending.

☆ OTHER SLEEP TIPS:

- Take naps when you can.
- Sleep with a sleep mask or darkened shades for the best night sleep
- Lavender oil can be sprayed on the sheets for relaxation
- Melatonin can help with sleep

FOOD

The food we eat can have an impact on symptoms in the body. There is much written about Anti-inflammatory type of foods, organic foods and some spices. There are also many diets based on gluten intake. Many of my friends and family who have eliminated gluten from their diets have seen their arthritic issues significantly improve. It would be to your advantage to research this for yourself.

I am a believer that fad diets are not a healthy way to live, but a change of lifestyle is healthy. In other words, change your overall eating regimen instead of trying fad diets. Here's the good news, you can change little by little over time. You don't have to change everything all on at once but changing your way of eating over time will ensure a healthier YOU. You will want to be the best decision maker for your change in the way you eat. I encourage you to do some research and choose a way of eating which fits your lifestyle. My only suggestion for a good overall diet is to investigate the Mediterranean diet. Other than this - decide what fits your tastes and needs best.

The relationship between inflammation and anti-inflammatory foods can have an impact on healing our body. I am learning more and more about how the health of our stomach has a direct affect on our overall well being. I encourage you to do your own research regarding probiotics and prebiotics, and learn how to help your stomach health through proper intake of foods overall. I am no expert in this field and I encourage you to do your own research however I have included the following foods/spices which help with reducing inflammation as well as foods which can inflame the body.

☆ FOODS WHICH REDUCE AND INCREASE INFLAMMATION

SPICES helpful for reducing inflammation:
Murik Cumann
Cinnamon
Tumeric

☆ FOODS HELPFUL FOR REDUCING INFLAMMATION:

Tomatoes
Olive Oil
Green Leafy Vegetables
Nuts: Almonds / Walnuts
Fatty Fish: Salmon / Tuna
Fruits: Blueberries / Cherries

☆ FOODS WHICH INFLAME THE BODY:

Refined Carbohydrates – white bread / sweets/ pastries
Fried Foods – French fries, etc.,
Soda
Red Meat- Processed Meats
Margarine / Shortening

SHOE WEAR

Believe it or not shoe wear is extremely important when dealing with a low back pain, especially with sciatica. You would do well and heal quicker in shoes which are made to give great support to your feet and therefore, the rest of your body.

☆ ABOUT THE SOLES:

The softer the sole, the more support given around your ankle and below your heel, the better off you are. My shoe of choice is **Nike Air**, but any good walking shoe with good support is great. You will want a shoe which can absorb some of the force as your heel strikes the ground. This will give you some relief, as your leg will not be absorbing as much force, which will ease the force into the low back as well.

☆ SHOES THAT COMPROMISE HEALING:

Hard soled shoes, high-heels, flip flops, ballet flats and mules are all very unsupportive shoes. These are not the best things to wear when dealing with sciatica or any type of back pain or foot pain. Think in terms of support and trying to take as much force off the heel as possible with every step. This will decrease the pressure going into the back.

ACTIVITIES OF DAILY LIVING

☆ DAILY ACTIVITIES:

Most people with sciatica and low back pain find it extremely painful to do simple daily activities such as brushing teeth, getting up-and-down from the toilet, placing things into a dishwasher or sink, reaching into cupboards and doing laundry. Any type of bending and lifting can be excruciating.

Whether you're pulling out drawers to get your clothes, or moving about the house, bending over to lift something can be a daunting task. Here is what typically happens when we lift or bend. We usually lift or bend from our low back with our feet aligned or in line with each other. This can be harmful to your muscles especially during the healing process.

☆ OVERALL HELPFUL TIPS FOR DAILY ACTIVITIES:

Here is what I tell my clients. Put the less painful leg in front of the more painful leg and bend from the waist. Bending like this will make your hips hinge properly and take pressure off of your low back.

☆ LOADING THE DISHWASHER / DOING LAUNDRY:

When loading a dishwasher, doing laundry or having to bend low, try to squat with both legs like a toddler squatting down -- not bending from the waist but rather squatting all the way down putting your buttocks to your heels. OR, if you have bad knees, you can stagger your feet as mentioned above so your painful leg is behind and your "good" leg is in front and bend from the waist, avoiding unwanted back strain.

☆ GETTING GROCERIES OUT OF THE CAR:

The best advice I can give is this: 1. Keep bags as close to your body as possible, so limit your reaching into the car seat or the trunk. This means move your body as close as possible before lifting and pulling the bags towards you. IF in a trunk, get as close as possible to lift the bags, which means plan ahead and put the bags as close to the edge of trunk as possible. Keeping the car clean can also save your clothes from getting dirty!

☆ WASHING DISHES/BRUSHING TEETH:

When using a sink for ANYTHING, instead of bending over from the waist, place a foot into the cupboard immediately below the sink to it causes you to hinge from your hips and allows your larger butt, and hip muscles to support you and NOT your back muscles.

☆ REACHING INTO CUPBOARDS:

Before reaching into cupboards for a glass or bowl or any item, check to see which arm is feels more comfortable when raising to the needed height. Again, get your body as close as possible to keep the item as close to your body as possible. Rreach with the more comfortable arm into cupboard.

☆ GETTING ON AND OFF THE TOILET:

This can be the trickiest one as houses are typically not equipped with a handicap bar or elevated seats, which would be very advantageous to have. Otherwise, IF the countertop or tub is not close to toilet, which you can use to push yourself up with, having a spouse/significant other help may be the only way to get off the pot ☹

☆ VACUUMING:

If and when vacuuming is needed, use your legs to move the vacuum, with NO reaching forward and pushing with your arms and trunk! This will take pressure and strain off your low back and allow your large leg and butt muscles to do more of the work.

POSITIONS

☆ AVOIDING PAINFUL POSITIONS:

My overall goal with patient education and treatments is to AVOID PAIN at all costs. Even though it may be totally impossible to **not** cause pain with certain activities, I tell my patients to avoid it as much as possible. Again, let's think of the letters "L M L." You can memorize this to help you think of "**L**ess Painful; **M**ore Comfortable; **L**ess Restrictive."

☆ COMPARABLE POSITIONS ON THE GOOD SIDE:

Initially I try to tell patients to find a comparable position which mimics the painful position on the bad side ---do this on the good side and maintain this position until it becomes uncomfortable. Then, move to another position you can get into which is comfortable initially even if it's only for 30 seconds to 5 minutes. Maintain this 2nd position until the position becomes uncomfortable. If you have a 3rd and 4th position which are comfortable this is great but just find 2 or more positions you know you can get into which are relatively comfortable compared to the normal pain. Rotate those 2,3 or 4 positions however often as needed to avoid flaring up.

☆ BODY BALANCE AND COMPENSATION:

You will notice over time, as you go from position to position (as stated above) the amount of time you can maintain a position before the pain starts getting really intense should increase. So even if you are in a position for a minute or two, you will be giving your body more of a chance to work and heal itself as well as to pump out excess fluid. This will minimize pain relax muscle spasms and compensatory spasms. Your body had likely been compensating due to the pain you have experienced. Think of this in terms of how your body naturally tries to balance itself. The body naturally tries to compensate to protect itself.

☆ MAINTAINING GOOD POSITION:

The goal for you is to find the most comfortable position mimicking the painful position and maintain it for as long as you can until it becomes uncomfortable. Get into your next position and continue doing that as often as needed to get to a position where the pain starts to calm down.

A FINAL NOTE

I HOPE YOU FOUND this information overview helpful. I have a passion to help people and to explain things in a quick, simple and concise manner. I feel everyone deserves to be able to have access to helpful and understandable information for their healthcare. My hope is you have learned some new ways to relieve and/or control your pain and this gets you started on Recovery Road. Feel free to contact me via email at info@SciaticaReliefNow.net.

Also, I would LOVE to have you join my Facebook group Sciatica & Piriformis Syndrome RELIEF Group (where it all started!). I also have a business FB page: Sciatica Relief Now.

I currently offer Sciatica Relief Now Group sites which have a small monthly fee to participate. IF interested, email me at info@SciaticaReliefNow.net, or visit my website for more information at www.SciaticaReliefNow.net. You can also watch many of the testimonials of people whom I have helped.

I also offer 1:1 Video Consultations with an Initial Consult free (I will keep doing this as long as time permits!). For more information you can email me at info@SciaticaReliefNow.net. To simply get more information, visit our website at www.SciaticaReliefNow.net.

ABOUT THE AUTHOR

DEAN VOLK IS an International Sciatica Consultant who LOVES to help those suffering from SCIATICA return to LIVING their LIVES WITHOUT PAIN pills, injections or surgery.

Dean, graduated with a Master of Physical Therapy from Northern Arizona University in 1992, and has been practicing for more than 25 years. He furthered his studies with numerous post-graduate courses focusing on the shoulder, knee, and back, with a strong emphasis in manual therapy. He completed courses in Total Motion Release (Levels 1, 2 and 3), which has afforded him an excellent way to relieve pain and restore function quickly and effectively.

With 25+ years of experience in Physical Therapy, Dean has practiced in various orthopedic and sports focused clinical settings, in Phoenix, AZ, Charlotte NC and now in Charleston SC. He opened his first NC clinic in 2006, and then expanded to a second facility in 2012. At the end of 2017, he started a small practice in Charleston, SC, and since mid-April 2018 has been working on Sciatica Relief Now.

Due to his love for helping those with Sciatica, Dean has established himself as an International Sciatica Consultant. He often holds Free Webinars on Sciatica which is attended by sufferers from all over the globe. He enjoys watching clients' faces as they start to move better, feel less pain and have HOPE RESTORED. His goal is to get people functioning normally by following very simple principles.

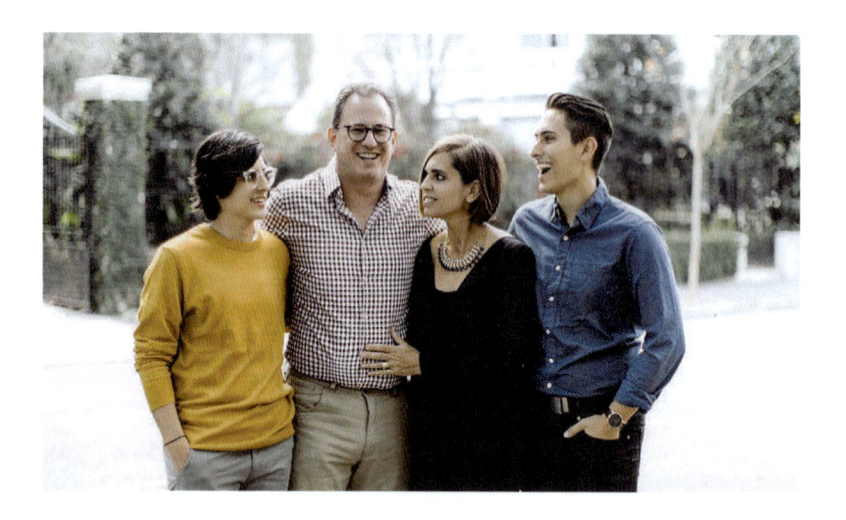

Dean and his wife, Trudy, have 2 sons, Ben and Jesse, both of whom graduated from College of Charleston. Dean is an avid AZ sports fan, enjoys spending time with his family and working with his clients to improve their lives.

Disclaimer

THIS BOOK IS for those dealing with sciatica issues. It is NOT a substitute or meant as a replacement for medical care by a local medical provider. This book does NOT diagnose or claim to diagnose or even heal any disease or condition. Before using the techniques in this book, you are advised to consult with your own physician or healthcare specialist regarding the suggestions and recommendations made in this book.

Neither the author, publisher, contributors, nor any other representatives will be liable for damages arising out of or in connection with the use of this book. This is a comprehensive limitation of liability which applies to all damages of any kind, including direct, indirect or consequential damages; loss of income, any injury or further damage to one's person, or any and all claims of third parties.

You understand this book is not intended as a substitute for consultation with a licensed healthcare practitioner, such as your physician. Before you begin any healthcare program, or change your lifestyle in any way, you will consult your physician or another licensed healthcare practitioner to ensure you are in good enough health and that the examples contained in this book will not harm you.

This book provides content related to physical health issues. As such, use of this book implies your acceptance of this disclaimer.

Printed in Great Britain
by Amazon